INTRODUCTION

Understand that Residue refers to material left in your digestive tract after the initial stages of digestion are finished. These materials often contain a lot of fiber because the body can't fully digest fiber. A low-residue diet is meant to put as few demands on the digestive tract as possible. The term 'residue' refers to any solid contents that end up in the large intestine after digestion. This includes undigested and unabsorbed food (which consists mostly of dietary fibre), bacteria, and gastric secretions. A low residue diet may help to prevent blockages in your bowel by reducing foods which are poorly or partially digested. The goal of a LRD is to decrease the size and frequency of bowel movements in order to reduce painful symptoms.

According to research made before writing this book, a low residue diet is recommended when people need to avoid foods that may irritate an inflamed bowel or block narrowed parts of the bowel. A low fibre diet may be one to recommend as a good option. When experiencing diarrhoea caused by a flare-up of inflammatory bowel disease such as Crohn's disease or ulcerative colitis - During a result of pelvic or abdominal radiotherapy - To prepare your bowel for investigations or surgery, according to "The Hillingdon Hospitals".

 Having a meal plan that puts as little demand on the digestive tract as possible is the logic behind a low-residue diet.You'll be able to integrate the diet to your preferred eating schedule, but the content and size of your meals will differ from what you're accustomed to.

The biggest change you'll be making on a low-residue diet is your fiber intake.

How does the low-residue diet work?

The low-residue diet has you consume no more than 10 to 15 grams of fiber every day. People without inflammatory bowel disease should ideally consume about 25 to 38 grams of fiber daily. You should also avoid dairy products and certain types of carbohydrates. They may provoke abdominal cramping and diarrhea. A doctor or dietitian should supervise you if you decide to follow a low-residue diet. People who follow this diet for too long may develop vitamin C and folic acid deficiencies. It can also change the gut bacteria. The amounts and types of food, as well as how long you follow the diet, should be dictated by your individual needs.

What is the difference between low residue diet and low fiber diet?

Both of them are quite resembling, except for the fact that a low-residue diet demands limiting the consumption of dairy products, so you wouldn't run the risk of increasing colonic residue and stool weight. The bottom line is that you'll give your gastrointestinal tract a much needed break.

Why eat a low residue diet?

Usually, physicians can prescribe this diet before or after certain medical procedures like colonoscopy, bowel surgery or in case of tumors or narrowing of the intestine. It may also be suggested to treat symptoms of irritable bowel syndrome, diverticulitis, diarrhea, Crohn's disease, ulcerative colitis. It's important to follow this diet precisely when it's prescribed, as it might cause unpleasant side effects and symptoms if you stick to it incorrectly.

Benefits of low residue diet

Reduce the bowel movements by cutting down on foods that are poorly digested

Reduce the amount of stool your body produces

Ease abdominal pain, diarrhea, and other symptoms

Ease the amount of work your digestive system isn't doing

How to follow a low-residue diet?

If your doctor recommends you to follow a low-residue diet, it would mean that you have to consume less vegetables, fruits, and grains. In some cases, doctors also advise avoiding milk and dairy products. Although milk doesn't contain fiber, it may cause discomfort, abdominal cramping, or diarrhea. However, your physician or nutritionist may prescribe you a diet, which would include more or less restrictions, depending on your medical condition and tolerance.

What You Can Eat

Grains

Refined or enriched white breads and plain crackers, such as saltines or Melba toast (no seeds)

Cooked cereals, like farina, cream of wheat, and grits

Cold cereals, like puffed rice and corn flakes

White rice, noodles, and refined pasta

Fruits and Vegetables

The skin and seeds of many fruits and vegetables are full of fiber, so you need to peel them and avoid the seeds.

These vegetables are OK:

Well-cooked fresh vegetables or canned vegetables without seeds, like asparagus tips, beets, green beans, carrots, mushrooms, spinach, squash (no seeds), and pumpkin

Cooked potatoes without skin

Tomato sauce (no seeds)

Fruits on the good list include:

Ripe bananas

Soft cantaloupe

Honeydew

Canned or cooked fruits without seeds or skin, like applesauce or canned pears

Avocado

Milk and Dairy

They're ok in moderation. Milk has no fiber, but it may trigger symptoms like diarrhea and cramping if you're lactose intolerant. If you are (meaning you have trouble processing dairy foods), you could take lactase supplements or buy lactose-free products.

Meats

Animal products don't have fiber. You can eat beef, lamb, chicken, fish (no bones), and pork, as long as they're lean, tender, and soft. Eggs are OK, too.

Fats, Sauces, and Condiments

These are all on the diet:

Margarine, butter, and oils

Mayonnaise and ketchup

Sour cream

Smooth sauces and salad dressing

Soy sauce

Clear jelly, honey, and syrup

Sweets and Snacks

You can satisfy your sweet tooth on a low-residue diet. These desserts and snacks are OK to eat in moderation:

Plain cakes and cookies

Gelatin, plain puddings, custard, and sherbet

Ice cream and ice pops

Hard candy

Pretzels (not whole-grain varieties)

Vanilla wafers

Drinks

Safe beverages include:

Decaffeinated coffee, tea, and carbonated beverages (caffeine can upset your stomach)

Milk

Juices made without seeds or pulp, like apple, no-pulp orange, and cranberry

Strained vegetable juices

What You Can't Eat

On this plan, you'll stay away from:

Coconut, seeds, and nuts, including those found in bread, cereal, desserts, and candy

Whole-grain products, including breads, cereals, crackers, pasta, rice, and kasha

Raw or dried fruits, like prunes, berries, raisins, figs, and pineapple

Most raw vegetables

Certain cooked vegetables, including peas, broccoli, winter squash, Brussels sprouts, cabbage, corn (and cornbread), onions, cauliflower, potatoes with skin, and baked

beans

Beans, lentils, and tofu

Tough meats with gristle, and smoked or cured deli meats

Cheese with seeds, nuts, or fruit

Crunchy peanut butter, jam, marmalade, and preserves

Pickles, olives, relish, sauerkraut, and horseradish

Popcorn

Fruit juices with pulp or seeds, prune juice, and pear nectar

How to Make It Work for You

As long as you follow the general guidelines for the diet, you can mix and match as much as you'd like. There are many meal options to choose from on a low-residue diet:

Breakfast

Decaffeinated coffee with cream and sugar

Cup of juice, such as no-pulp orange juice, apple juice, or cranberry juice

Farina

Scrambled eggs

Waffles, French toast, or pancakes

White-bread toast with margarine and grape jelly (no seeds)

Lunch

Baked chicken, white rice, canned carrots, or green beans

Salad with baked chicken, American cheese, smooth salad dressing, white dinner roll

Baked potato (no skin) with sour cream and butter or margarine

Hamburger with white seedless bun, ketchup, and mayonnaise -- and lettuce if it doesn't make your symptoms worse.

Dinner

Tender roast beef, white rice, cooked carrots or spinach, white dinner roll with margarine or butter

Pasta with butter or olive oil, French bread, fruit cocktail

Baked chicken, white rice or baked potato without skin, and cooked green beans

Broiled fish, white rice, and canned green beans

Does research support low-residue diets?

There is not a lot of recent research to support using a solid low-residue diet. There is more evidence to support using a short-term liquid, semi-elemental, and low-residue diet to manage symptoms of Crohn's disease. This diet consists only of nutritional shakes you can get from your doctor. Some doctors may recommend a solid low-residue diet to help manage acute symptoms.

A semi-elemental diet can effectively:

Improve absorption of nutrients

Increase weight and growth in malnourished children

Induce remission of symptoms

This diet can also function as an elimination diet. After you have been on the semi-elemental diet for a while, you may try slowly reintroducing foods. This will help you identify and exclude problematic foods. The LOFFLEX diet, or low fat/fiber limited exclusion diet, is similar and may also be recommended by your doctor.

Crohn's is a condition that affects everyone differently. This makes it difficult to prescribe one type of diet plan. In fact, your symptoms may vary over time. However, there is a significant amount of gut bacteria research that supports a high-fiber, plant-based diet for the prevention of inflammatory bowel disease and other digestive conditions.

Things to keep in mind

Fruits, vegetables, grains, and legumes supply important antioxidants, phytonutrients, vitamins, minerals, and other nutrients. Try to consume a balanced diet, as the low-residue diet may not provide enough vitamin C, folic acid, calcium, or antioxidants, or nutrients for gut bacteria, for example. All of these nutrients are essential for good health. Supplements may be necessary to correct dietary deficiencies.

Multiple diets are being studied for their potential benefit for inflammatory bowel diseases. These include the low-

FODMAP diet, plant-based diets, exclusion diets, and the LOFFLEX diet. Doctors don't recommend any one diet for everyone with Crohn's disease because the condition affects everyone differently. Consider consulting with a dietitian if you have any questions or concerns, or to help you individualize your nutrition approach.

RECIPES FOR LOW RESIDUE DIET

Guacamole

Ingredients

3 avocados - peeled, pitted, and mashed

1 lime, juiced

1 teaspoon salt

½ cup diced onion

3 tablespoons chopped fresh cilantro

2 roma (plum) tomatoes, diced

1 teaspoon minced garlic

1 pinch ground cayenne pepper (optional)

Directions

Step 1

In a medium bowl, mash together the avocados, lime juice, and salt. Mix in onion, cilantro, tomatoes, and garlic. Stir in cayenne pepper. Refrigerate 1 hour for 1best flavor, or serve immediately.

Nutrition Facts Per Serving:

262 calories; 22.2 g total fat; 0 mg cholesterol; 596 mg sodium. 18 g carbohydrates; 3.7 g protein

Garlic Prime Rib

Ingredients

1 (10 pound) prime rib roast

10 cloves garlic, minced

2 tablespoons olive oil

2 teaspoons salt

2 teaspoons ground black pepper

2 teaspoons dried thyme

Directions

Step 1

Place the roast in a roasting pan with the fatty side up. In a small bowl, mix together the garlic, olive oil, salt, pepper and thyme. Spread the mixture over the fatty layer of the roast, and let the roast sit out until it is at room temperature, no longer than 1 hour.

Step 2

Preheat the oven to 500 degrees F (260 degrees C).

Step 3

Bake the roast for 20 minutes in the preheated oven, then reduce the temperature to 325 degrees F (165 degrees C), and continue roasting for an additional 60 to 75 minutes. The internal temperature of the roast should be at 135 degrees F (57 degrees C) for medium rare.

Step 4

Allow the roast to rest for 10 or 15 minutes before carving so the meat can retain its juices.

Nutrition Facts Per Serving:

562 calories; 48 g total fat; 113 mg cholesterol; 395 mg sodium. 1 g carbohydrates; 29.6 g protein

Rosemary Roasted Turkey

Ingredients

¾ cup olive oil

3 tablespoons minced garlic

2 tablespoons chopped fresh rosemary

1 tablespoon chopped fresh basil

1 tablespoon Italian seasoning

1 teaspoon ground black pepper

salt to taste

1 (12 pound) whole turkey

Directions

Step 1

Preheat oven to 325 degrees F (165 degrees C).

Step 2

In a small bowl, mix the olive oil, garlic, rosemary, basil, Italian seasoning, black pepper and salt. Set aside.

Step 3

Wash the turkey inside and out; pat dry. Remove any large fat deposits. Loosen the skin from the breast. This is done by slowly working your fingers between the breast and the skin. Work it loose to the end of the drumstick, being careful not to tear the skin.

Step 4

Using your hand, spread a generous amount of the rosemary mixture under the breast skin and down the thigh and leg. Rub the remainder of the rosemary mixture over the outside of the breast. Use toothpicks to seal skin over any exposed breast meat.

Step 5

Place the turkey on a rack in a roasting pan. Add about 1/4 inch of water to the bottom of the pan. Roast in the preheated oven 3 to 4 hours, or until the internal temperature of the bird reaches 180 degrees F (80 degrees C).

Nutrition Facts Per Serving:

596 calories; 33.7 g total fat; 198 mg cholesterol; 165 mg sodium. 0.8 g carbohydrates; 68.1 g protein

Marinated Grilled Shrimp

Ingredients

3 cloves garlic, minced

⅓ cup olive oil

¼ cup tomato sauce

2 tablespoons red wine vinegar

2 tablespoons chopped fresh basil

½ teaspoon salt

¼ teaspoon cayenne pepper

2 pounds fresh shrimp, peeled and deveined

6 eaches skewers

Direction

Step 1

In a large bowl, stir together the garlic, olive oil, tomato sauce, and red wine vinegar. Season with basil, salt, and cayenne pepper. Add shrimp to the bowl, and stir until evenly coated. Cover, and refrigerate for 30 minutes to 1 hour, stirring once or twice.

Step 2

Preheat grill for medium heat. Thread shrimp onto skewers, piercing once near the tail and once near the head. Discard marinade.

Step 3

Lightly oil grill grate. Cook shrimp on preheated grill for 2 to 3 minutes per side, or until opaque.

Nutrition Facts Per Serving:

273 calories; 31 g protein; 2.8 g carbohydrates; 230 mg cholesterol; 471.8 mg sodium.

Foolproof Rib Roast

Ingredients

1 (5 pound) standing beef rib roast

2 teaspoons salt

1 teaspoon ground black pepper

1 teaspoon garlic powder

Directions

Step 1

Allow roast to stand at room temperature for at least 1 hour.

Step 2

Preheat the oven to 375 degrees F (190 degrees C). Combine the salt, pepper and garlic powder in a small cup. Place the roast on a rack in a roasting pan so that the fatty side is up and the rib side is on the bottom. Rub the seasoning onto the roast.

Step 3

Roast for 1 hour in the preheated oven. Turn the oven off and leave the roast inside. Do not open the door. Leave it in there for 3 hours. 30 to 40 minutes before serving, turn the oven back on at 375 degrees F (190 degrees C) to reheat the roast. The internal temperature should be at least 145 degrees F (62 degrees C). Remove from the oven and let rest for 10 minutes before carving into servings.

Nutrition Facts Per Serving:

576.1 calories; 37 g protein; 0.6 g carbohydrates; 137.2 mg cholesterol; 879.6 mg sodium.

Spinach and Feta Pita Bake

Ingredients

1 (6 ounce) tub sun-dried tomato pesto

6 (6 inch) whole wheat pita breads

2 roma (plum) tomatoes, chopped

1 bunch spinach, rinsed and chopped

4 fresh mushrooms, sliced

½ cup crumbled feta cheese

2 tablespoons grated Parmesan cheese

3 tablespoons olive oil

ground black pepper to taste

Directions

Step 1

Preheat the oven to 350 degrees F (175 degrees C).

Step 2

Spread tomato pesto onto one side of each pita bread and place them pesto-side up on a baking sheet. Top pitas with tomatoes, spinach, mushrooms, feta cheese, and Parmesan cheese; drizzle with olive oil and season with pepper.

Step 3

Bake in the preheated oven until pita breads are crisp, about 12 minutes. Cut pitas into quarters.

Nutrition Facts Per Serving:

350 calories; 17.1 g total fat; 13 mg cholesterol; 587 mg sodium. 41.6 g carbohydrates; 11.6 g protein;

Juicy Roasted Chicken

Ingredients

1 (3 pound) whole chicken, giblets removed

1 teaspoon salt and black pepper to taste

1 tablespoon onion powder, or to taste

½ cup margarine, divided

1 stalk celery, leaves removed

Directions

Step 1

Preheat oven to 350 degrees F (175 degrees C).

Step 2

Place chicken in a roasting pan, and season generously inside and out with salt and pepper. Sprinkle inside and out with onion powder. Place 3 tablespoons margarine in the chicken cavity. Arrange dollops of the remaining margarine around the chicken's exterior. Cut the celery into 3 or 4 pieces, and place in the chicken cavity.

Step 3

Bake uncovered 1 hour and 15 minutes in the preheated oven, to a minimum internal temperature of 180 degrees F (82 degrees C). Remove from heat, and baste with melted margarine and drippings. Cover with aluminum foil, and allow to rest about 30 minutes before serving.

Nutrition Facts Per Serving:

423.1 calories; 30.9 g protein; 1.2 g carbohydrates; 97 mg cholesterol; 661.9 mg sodium.

Simple Roasted Butternut Squash

Ingredients

1 butternut squash - peeled, seeded, and cut into 1-inch cubes

2 tablespoons olive oil

2 cloves garlic, minced

salt and ground black pepper to taste

Directions

Step 1

Preheat oven to 400 degrees F (200 degrees C).

Step 2

Toss butternut squash with olive oil and garlic in a large bowl. Season with salt and black pepper. Arrange coated squash on a baking sheet.

Step 3

Roast in the preheated oven until squash is tender and lightly browned, 25 to 30 minutes.

Nutrition Facts Per Serving:

177 calories; 7 g total fat; 0 mg cholesterol; 11 mg sodium. 30.3 g carbohydrates; 2.6 g protein

Roast Sticky Chicken-Rotisserie

Ingredients

4 teaspoons salt

2 teaspoons paprika

1 teaspoon onion powder

1 teaspoon dried thyme

1 teaspoon white pepper

½ teaspoon cayenne pepper

½ teaspoon black pepper

½ teaspoon garlic powder

2 onions, quartered

2 (4 pound) whole chickens

Directions

Step 1

In a small bowl, mix together salt, paprika, onion powder, thyme, white pepper, black pepper, cayenne pepper, and garlic powder. Remove and discard giblets from chicken. Rinse chicken cavity, and pat dry with paper towel. Rub each chicken inside and out with spice mixture. Place 1 onion into the cavity of each chicken. Place chickens in a resealable bag or double wrap with plastic wrap. Refrigerate overnight, or at least 4 to 6 hours.

Step 2

Preheat oven to 250 degrees F (120 degrees C).

Step 3

Place chickens in a roasting pan. Bake uncovered for 5 hours, to a minimum internal temperature of 180 degrees F (85 degrees C). Let the chickens stand for 10 minutes before carving.

Nutrition Facts Per Serving:

585.7 calories; 61.7 g protein; 3.7 g carbohydrates; 194.1 mg cholesterol; 1350.8 mg sodium.

Cajun Spice Mix

Ingredients

   2 teaspoons salt

   2 teaspoons garlic powder

   2 ½ teaspoons paprika

   1 teaspoon ground black pepper

   1 teaspoon onion powder

   1 teaspoon cayenne pepper

   1 ¼ teaspoons dried oregano

   1 ¼ teaspoons dried thyme

   ½ teaspoon red pepper flakes (optional)

Directions

Step 1

Stir together salt, garlic powder, paprika, black pepper, onion powder, cayenne pepper, oregano, thyme, and red pepper flakes until evenly blended. Store in an airtight container.

Nutrition Facts Per Serving:

6 calories; 0.1 g total fat; 0 mg cholesterol; 388 mg sodium. 1.2 g carbohydrates; 0.2 g protein

Grilled Asparagus

Ingredients

1 pound fresh asparagus spears, trimmed

1 tablespoon olive oil

salt and pepper to taste

Directions

Step 1

Preheat grill for high heat.

Step 2

Lightly coat the asparagus spears with olive oil. Season with salt and pepper to taste.

Step 3

Grill over high heat for 2 to 3 minutes, or to desired tenderness.

Nutrition Facts Per Serving:

53 calories; 3.5 g total fat; 0 mg cholesterol; 2 mg sodium. 4.4 g carbohydrates; 2.5 g protein

Ken's Perfect Hard Boiled Egg

Ingredient

1 tablespoon salt

¼ cup distilled white vinegar

6 cups water

8 eggs

Directions

Step 1

Combine the salt, vinegar, and water in a large pot, and bring to a boil over high heat. Add the eggs one at a time, being careful not to crack them. Reduce the heat to a gentle boil, and cook for 14 minutes.

Step 2

Once the eggs have cooked, remove them from the hot water, and place into a container of ice water or cold, running water. Cool completely, about 15 minutes. Store in the refrigerator up to 1 week.

Nutrition Facts Per Serving:

71.7 calories; 6.3 g protein; 0. 4 g carbohydrates; 186 mg cholesterol; 947.4 mg sodium.

Spinach and Feta Pita Bake

Ingredients

1 (6 ounce) tub sun-dried tomato pesto

6 (6 inch) whole wheat pita breads

2 plum tomato (blank)s roma (plum) tomatoes, chopped

1 bunch spinach, rinsed and chopped

4 medium (blank)s fresh mushrooms, sliced

½ cup crumbled feta cheese

2 tablespoons grated Parmesan cheese

3 tablespoons olive oil

1 pinch ground black pepper to taste

Directions

Step 1

Preheat the oven to 350 degrees F (175 degrees C).

Step 2

Spread tomato pesto onto one side of each pita bread and place them pesto-side up on a baking sheet. Top pitas with tomatoes, spinach, mushrooms, feta cheese, and Parmesan cheese; drizzle with olive oil and season with pepper.

Step 3

Bake in the preheated oven until pita breads are crisp, about 12 minutes. Cut pitas into quarters.

Nutrition Facts Per Serving:

349.9 calories; protein 11.6g 23% DV; carbohydrates 41.6g 13% DV; fat 17.1g 26% DV; cholesterol 12.6mg 4% DV; sodium 587.1mg 24% DV.

Greek God Pasta

Ingredients

1 (16 ounce) package whole wheat rotini pasta

1 (16 ounce) can peeled and diced tomatoes, drained

2 tablespoons chopped green bell pepper

¼ cup chopped green onion

3 cups tomato sauce

1 teaspoon dried basil

1 teaspoon dried oregano

1 cup sliced black olives

½ cup shredded mozzarella cheese

2 tablespoons crumbled feta cheese

Directions

Step 1

Preheat the oven to 400 degrees F (200 degrees C).

Step 2

Bring a large pot of lightly salted water to a boil. Add rotini pasta, and cook until al dente, about 8 minutes. Drain and pour into a deep casserole dish.

Step 3

Stir tomatoes, green pepper, green onion, olives and tomato sauce into the pasta. Season with basil and oregano and mix until evenly blended. Sprinkle mozzarella and feta cheese over the top.

Step 4

Bake for 30 minutes in the preheated oven, until cheese is melted and bubbly. Let stand for a few minutes before serving.

Nutrition Facts Per Serving:

371.4 calories; protein 16.4g 33% DV; carbohydrates 68.5g 22% DV; fat 6g 9% DV; cholesterol 8.8mg 3% DV; sodium 1068.1mg 43% DV.

Spinach-Feta Casserole

Ingredients

2 (10 ounce) packages frozen chopped spinach

8 ounces crumbled feta cheese

2 cups shredded mozzarella cheese

1 cup cubed processed cheese food

1 cup melted butter, divided

2 tablespoons distilled white vinegar

½ teaspoon garlic powder

salt and pepper to taste

1 (16 ounce) package phyllo dough

Directions

Step 1

Preheat oven to 425 degrees F (220 degrees C).

Step 2

In a large bowl, combine the spinach, feta cheese, mozzarella cheese, processed cheese food, 1/2 the butter, vinegar, garlic powder, salt and pepper. Mix well and set aside.

Step 3

Place a layer of phyllo dough into the bottom of a lightly greased 2-quart casserole dish. Spread the spinach and cheese mixture into the dish and top with 4 layers of phyllo dough, spraying each layer with butter-flavored cooking spray. Drizzle the remaining butter over the top.

Step 4

Bake at 425 degrees F (220 degrees C) for 20 minutes.

Nutrition Facts Per Serving:

547.7 calories; protein 18.6g 37% DV; carbohydrates 31.8g 10% DV; fat 37.7g 58% DV; cholesterol 108.4mg 36% DV; sodium 1164.1mg 47% DV.

Spanakopita (Greek Spinach Pie)

Ingredients

   3 tablespoons olive oil

   1 large onion, chopped

   1 bunch green onions, chopped

   2 cloves garlic, minced

   2 pounds spinach, rinsed and chopped

   ½ cup chopped fresh parsley

   2 large eggs eggs, lightly beaten

   ½ cup ricotta cheese

   1 cup crumbled feta cheese

   8 sheets phyllo dough

   ¼ cup olive oil

Directions

   Step 1

Preheat oven to 350 degrees F (175 degrees C). Lightly oil a 9x9 inch square baking pan.

Step 2

Heat 3 tablespoons olive oil in a large skillet over medium heat. Saute onion, green onions and garlic, until soft and lightly browned. Stir in spinach and parsley, and continue to saute until spinach is limp, about 2 minutes. Remove from heat and set aside to cool.

Step 3

In a medium bowl, mix together eggs, ricotta, and feta. Stir in spinach mixture. Lay 1 sheet of phyllo dough in prepared baking pan, and brush lightly with olive oil. Lay another sheet of phyllo dough on top, brush with olive oil, and repeat process with two more sheets of phyllo. The sheets will overlap the pan. Spread spinach and cheese mixture into pan and fold overhanging dough over filling. Brush with oil, then layer remaining 4 sheets of phyllo dough, brushing each with oil. Tuck overhanging dough into pan to seal filling.

Step 4

Bake in preheated oven for 30 to 40 minutes, until golden brown. Cut into squares and serve while hot.

Nutrition Facts Per Serving:

494.1 calories; protein 18.2g 36% DV; carbohydrates 31.5g 10% DV; fat 34.7g 53% DV; cholesterol 100.3mg 33% DV; sodium 893.9mg 36% DV.

A Lot More Than Plain Spinach Pie (Greek Batsaria)

Ingredient

  3 large eggs eggs

  1 pound chopped fresh spinach

  3 leeks leeks, chopped

  5 eaches green onions, chopped

2 ⅓ cups crumbled feta cheese

1 bunch parsley, chopped

1 bunch dill, chopped

1 bunch spearmint, chopped

1 teaspoon white sugar

1 cup milk

¾ cup olive oil

1 pinch salt and ground black pepper to taste

2 ½ cups all-purpose flour

½ cup semolina flour

1 pinch salt

¼ cup olive oil

2 cups water

1 ¼ cups grated Parmesan cheese

2 tablespoons cold butter, cut into pieces

2 tablespoons olive oil

Directions

Step 1

Preheat an oven to 350 degrees F (175 degrees C). Grease a deep 9x9 inch baking dish.

Step 2

Beat the eggs in a mixing bowl, then stir in the spinach, leeks, green onions, feta cheese, parsley, dill, spearmint, sugar, milk, and 3/4 cup of olive oil until evenly mixed. Season to taste with salt and pepper; set aside. Whisk together the all-purpose flour, semolina flour, and 1 pinch of salt in a mixing bowl. Stir in 1/4 cup of olive oil and the water until no lumps remain. Pour 2/3 of the batter into the prepared 9x9 inch pan, and spread out evenly. Spoon the spinach filling over the batter, then spoon the remaining batter overtop. Sprinkle with the Parmesan cheese, butter pieces, and 2 tablespoons of olive oil.

Step 3

Bake in the preheated oven until the bottom crust and top has firmed and nicely browned, about 1 hour.

Nutrition Facts Per Serving:

649.8 calories; protein 20.1g 40% DV; carbohydrates 45g 15% DV; fat 44.1g 68% DV; cholesterol 115.3mg 38% DV; sodium 714.2mg 29% DV.

Pico de Gallo

Ingredients

6 plum tomato (blank)s roma (plum) tomatoes, diced

½ red onion, minced

3 tablespoons chopped fresh cilantro

½ jalapeno pepper, seeded and minced

½ lime, juiced

1 clove garlic, minced

1 pinch garlic powder

1 pinch ground cumin, or to taste

1 pinch salt and ground black pepper to taste

Directions

Step 1

Stir the tomatoes, onion, cilantro, jalapeno pepper, lime juice, garlic, garlic powder, cumin, salt, and pepper together in a bowl. Refrigerate at least 3 hours before serving.

Nutrition Facts Per Serving:

9.6 calories; protein 0.4g 1% DV; carbohydrates 2.2g 1% DV; fat 0.1g; cholesterolmg; sodium 15.2mg 1% DV.

Farm-to-Table Pico de Gallo

Ingredients

4 medium (blank)s Roma (plum) tomatoes, diced

1 cup diced onion

1 carrot, peeled and chopped

¼ cup fresh cilantro leaves, or to taste

3 small jalapeno peppers

2 eaches green chile peppers

¼ large poblano chile

1 lime, juiced

1 tablespoon chopped garlic

1 teaspoon sea salt

Directions

Step 1

Mix tomatoes and onion in a bowl.

Step 2

Process carrot, cilantro, jalapeno peppers, green chile peppers, poblano chile, lime juice, and garlic in a food processor to your preferred texture; add to tomato mixture and stir. Season the mixture with sea salt.

Step 3

Cover bowl with plastic wrap and refrigerate at least 2 hours before serving.

Nutrition Facts Per Serving:

27.1 calories; protein 1g 2% DV; carbohydrates 6.2g 2% DV; fat 0.2g; cholesterolmg; sodium 230.6mg 9% DV.

Cabbage Pico de Gallo

Ingredients

1 medium head cabbage, chopped

6 medium (blank)s Roma (plum) tomatoes, diced

1 red onion, diced

1 yellow onion, diced

4 medium (blank)s jalapeno peppers, diced

2 bunches cilantro, chopped

3 lime (2" dia)s limes, juiced

2 teaspoons chopped garlic

2 teaspoons salt

Directions

Step 1

Mix cabbage, tomatoes, red onion, yellow onion, jalapeno pepper, cilantro, lime juice, garlic, and salt in a large bowl.

Step 2

Cover bowl with plastic wrap and refrigerate at least 2 hours.

Nutrition Facts Per Serving:

27 calories; protein 1.2g 2% DV; carbohydrates 6.5g 2% DV; fat 0.2g; cholesterolmg; sodium 245.2mg 10% DV.

Secret Ingredient Pico de Gallo

Ingredients

½ cup minced onion

2 peppers jalapeno peppers, seeded and minced

¼ cup diced red bell pepper

¼ cup minced dill pickle

4 large tomatoes, seeded and diced

1 tablespoon fresh lime juice

¼ cup chopped cilantro

1 pinch salt and pepper to taste

Directions

Step 1

In a medium bowl, combine the onion, jalapeno pepper, bell pepper, dill pickle, and diced tomatoes. Stir in lime juice and cilantro; season to taste with salt and pepper. Cover, and refrigerate at least 1 hour before serving, preferably overnight.

Nutrition Facts Per Serving:

49.5 calories; protein 2.2g 4% DV; carbohydrates 10.9g 4% DV; fat 0.5g 1% DV; cholesterolmg; sodium 126.4mg 5% DV.

Scott's Pico de Gallo

Ingredients

   3 large tomatoes, diced

   1 white onion, diced

   1 bunch cilantro, chopped

   6 fruit (2" dia)s limes, juiced

   1 tablespoon salt, or to taste

Directions

Step 1

Toss tomatoes, white onion, and cilantro together in a large bowl. Pour lime juice over tomato mixture; mix to coat. Season with salt. Chill completely before serving.

Nutrition Facts Per Serving:

34.5 calories; protein 1.3g 3% DV; carbohydrates 9.5g 3% DV; fat 0.3g; cholesterolmg; sodium 880.2mg 35% DV.

Juicy Roasted Chicken

Ingredients

1 (3 pound) whole chicken, giblets removed

1 teaspoon salt and black pepper to taste

1 tablespoon onion powder, or to taste

½ cup margarine, divided

1 stalk celery, leaves removed

Directions

Step 1

Preheat oven to 350 degrees F (175 degrees C).

Step 2

Place chicken in a roasting pan, and season generously inside and out with salt and pepper. Sprinkle inside and out with onion powder. Place 3 tablespoons margarine in the chicken cavity. Arrange dollops of the remaining margarine around the chicken's exterior. Cut the celery into 3 or 4 pieces, and place in the chicken cavity.

Step 3

Bake uncovered 1 hour and 15 minutes in the preheated oven, to a minimum internal temperature of 180 degrees F (82 degrees C). Remove from heat, and baste with melted margarine and drippings. Cover with aluminum foil, and allow to rest about 30 minutes before serving.

Nutrition Facts Per Serving:

423.1 calories; protein 30.9g 62% DV; carbohydrates 1.2g; fat 32.1g 49% DV; cholesterol 97mg 32% DV; sodium 661.9mg 27% DV.

Crispy Roasted Chicken

Ingredients

1 teaspoon kosher salt

½ teaspoon caraway seeds

½ teaspoon dried sage

¼ teaspoon fennel seeds

¼ teaspoon coriander seeds

¼ teaspoon dried rosemary

2 tablespoons paprika

2 teaspoons garlic powder

2 teaspoons all-purpose flour

1 teaspoon onion powder

5 tablespoons vegetable oil

1 (4 pound) broiler-fryer chicken, cut in half lengthwise

Directions

Step 1

Preheat oven to 425 degrees F (220 degrees C).

Step 2

In a spice grinder or mortar, combine kosher salt, caraway seeds, sage, fennel, coriander, and rosemary. Grind to a coarse powder. Transfer spice mixture to a bowl and stir in paprika, garlic powder, flour, and onion powder; mix in vegetable oil to make a smooth paste.

Step 3

Pat chicken halves dry with paper towels and tuck wing tips up behind the back. Brush spice paste onto chicken halves, coating both sides, taking care to season under wings and legs. Place chicken halves in baking dish or roasting pan with skin sides up, leaving space around chicken so halves aren't touching.

Step 4

Roast in preheated oven until a thermometer inserted in a thigh reads 165 degrees F (74 degrees C), about 1 hour. Remove from oven and let rest for 10 minutes before slicing.

Nutrition Facts Per Serving:

495.3 calories; protein 41.5g 83% DV; carbohydrates 3.1g 1% DV; fat 34.5g 53% DV; cholesterol 129.3mg 43% DV; sodium 445.6mg 18% DV.

German Chicken

Ingredients

4 breast half, bone and skin removed (blank)s skinless, boneless chicken breast halves

1 cup barbecue sauce

22 ounces sauerkraut

Directions

Step 1

Preheat oven to 350 degrees F (175 degrees C).

Step 2

In a 9x13 inch baking dish, place the sauerkraut in a single layer. Place the chicken breasts on top of the sauerkraut. Pour the barbecue sauce over the chicken. Cover and bake in the preheated oven for 30 minutes or until the chicken is cooked and the juices run clear.

Nutrition Facts Per Serving:

252.8 calories; protein 28.6g 57% DV; carbohydrates 29.2g 9% DV; fat 1.9g 3% DV; cholesterol 68.4mg 23% DV; sodium 1794mg 72% DV.

Roast Duck with Chestnut Stuffing

Ingredients

  1 onion, peeled and cut into chunks

  1 parsley root, peeled and cut into chunks

  1 carrot, roughly chopped

  1 sprig fresh rosemary

  2 leaf (blank)s bay leaves

  1 teaspoon whole white peppercorns

  2 cups dry white wine

  1 whole duck

Stuffing:

  2 cups finely chopped roasted chestnuts

  1 apple, peeled and finely chopped

  2 slices bread, diced

  1 egg

1 teaspoon dried tarragon, or to taste

1 pinch salt and freshly ground pepper to taste

wooden skewers

2 tablespoons rapeseed oil, or more if needed

Directions

Step 1

Combine onion, parsley root, carrot, rosemary, bay leaves, and white peppercorns in a bowl. Stir in white wine. Place duck in a large bowl and pour marinade over duck. Cover with foil and marinate in the fridge for at least 12 hours.

Step 2

Preheat oven to 425 degrees F (220 degrees C).

Step 3

Combine chestnuts, apple, bread, and egg in a bowl; season with tarragon, salt, and pepper.

Step 4

Remove duck from the marinade and strain marinade through a sieve. Dry duck inside and out with paper towels. Rub salt and pepper all over the skin. Fill cavity with stuffing, being careful not to overstuff. Secure opening with wooden skewers. Pour oil into a roasting dish. Add stuffed duck, breast-side up.

Step 5

Roast duck in the preheated oven, turning occasionally, until golden brown on all sides, about 20 minutes.

Step 6

Heat marinade in a saucepan over medium heat until warmed through, about 5 minutes.

Step 7

Pour warm marinade into the roasting pan. Cover with a lid or aluminum foil and return to the oven. Reduce oven temperature to 350 degrees F (175 degrees C) and bake duck until no longer pink at the bone and the juices run clear, about 90 minutes. An instant-read thermometer inserted into the thickest part of the thigh, near the bone, should read 165 degrees F (74 degrees C).

Step 8

Remove duck from the roasting pan and transfer to a baking sheet. Set oven rack about 6 inches from the heat source and preheat the oven's broiler. Roast duck until skin is golden-brown, 3 to 5 minutes. Remove duck from the oven, cover with a doubled sheet of aluminum foil, and allow to rest in a warm area for 10 minutes before slicing.

Step 9

Strain the stock, removing any burnt bits and skimming off fat. Heat stock in a saucepan over high heat and cook until gravy is reduced to 1/3, 5 to 10 minutes. Season with salt and pepper. Carve duck and serve with gravy.

Nutrition Facts Per Serving:

302.2 calories; protein 7.2g 14% DV; carbohydrates 36g 12% DV; fat 8g 12% DV; cholesterol 47.2mg 16% DV; sodium 132.1mg 5% DV.

Grillhaxe (Grilled Eisbein, Pork Shanks)

Ingredients

1 cup olive oil

2 tablespoons dried marjoram

2 tablespoons dried basil

2 tablespoons chopped fresh thyme

2 tablespoons chopped fresh rosemary

2 tablespoons sea salt

1 teaspoon paprika

1 teaspoon ground black pepper

1 teaspoon vegetable bouillon powder

6 (1 1/2) pounds pork shanks

Directions

Step 1

Preheat oven to 350 degrees F (175 degrees C).

Step 2

Whisk olive oil, marjoram, basil, rosemary, thyme, sea salt, paprika, black pepper, and vegetable bouillon powder together in a bowl. Rub pork shanks with herb rub and arrange on a large baking pan.

Step 3

Roast in preheated oven until shanks are tender and outer skin is crispy, about 3 hours.

Nutrition Facts Per Serving:

532.3 calories; protein 70.6g 141% DV; carbohydrates 0.8g; fat 27.9g 43% DV; cholesterol 185.9mg 62% DV; sodium 3080.5mg 123% DV.

Baked Chicken Wings

Ingredients

    3 tablespoons olive oil

    3 cloves garlic, pressed

    2 teaspoons chili powder

    1 teaspoon garlic powder

    1 pinch salt and ground black pepper to taste

    10 eaches chicken wings

Directions

    Step 1

    Preheat the oven to 375 degrees F (190 degrees C).

    Step 2

Combine the olive oil, garlic, chili powder, garlic powder, salt, and pepper in a large, resealable bag; seal and shake to combine. Add the chicken wings; reseal and shake to coat. Arrange the chicken wings on a baking sheet.

Step 3

Cook the wings in the preheated oven 1 hour, or until crisp and cooked through.

Nutrition Facts Per Serving:

532.1 calories; protein 31.7g 64% DV; carbohydrates 3.9g 1% DV; fat 43.1g 66% DV; cholesterol 96.6mg 32% DV; sodium 122.6mg 5% DV.

Lemon Pepper Chicken Wings

Ingredients

6 tablespoons olive oil

¼ cup finely grated lemon zest

2 tablespoons coarse sea salt

2 tablespoons ground black pepper

1 (3 pound) bag chicken wings

Directions

Step 1

Preheat oven to 425 degrees F (220 degrees C). Line a baking sheet with parchment paper.

Step 2

Whisk olive oil, lemon zest, salt, and black pepper together in a bowl; add wings and toss to coat. Spread coated wings in a single layer onto the prepared baking sheet.

Step 3

Bake in the preheated oven until no longer pink at the bone and the juices run clear, about 35 minutes. An instant-read thermometer inserted near the bone should read 165 degrees F (74 degrees C). Bake longer for a crispier skin.

Nutrition Facts Per Serving:

291 calories; protein 15.5g 31% DV; carbohydrates 2g 1% DV; fat 24.6g 38% DV; cholesterol 47.6mg 16% DV; sodium 1807.9mg 72% DV.

Baked Sticky Chicken Wings

Ingredients

10 eaches chicken wings, separated at joints, tips discarded

1 pinch salt to taste

1 cup mayonnaise

1 cup peach chutney

1 (1.25 ounce) envelope dry onion soup mix

2 cups hot water

Directions

Step 1

Preheat the oven to 350 degrees F (175 degrees C).

Step 2

Place the chicken wings in a roasting pan. Season with salt. In a medium bowl, stir together the mayonnaise, peach chutney, onion soup mix and hot water. Pour this over the chicken wings.

Step 3

Bake in the preheated oven until the sauce is brown and sticky, about 1 hour and 15 minutes.

Nutrition Facts Per Serving:

689.6 calories, protein 17.4g 35% DV; carbohydrates 34g 11% DV; fat 55.4g 85% DV; cholesterol 69.2mg 23% DV; sodium 1186mg 47% DV.

Easy Lemon Pepper Chicken Wings

Ingredients

2 cups oil, or as needed

2 tablespoons extra-virgin olive oil

1 tablespoon lemon pepper seasoning (such as McCormick®)

12 eaches chicken wings

Directions

Step 1

Heat oil in a deep-fryer or large saucepan to 375 degrees F (190 degrees C).

Step 2

Stir olive oil and lemon pepper together in a bowl.

Step 3

Fry the chicken wings in hot oil until no longer pink at the bone and the juices run clear, about 8 minutes. An instant-read thermometer inserted near the bone should read 165 degrees F (74 degrees C).

Step 4

Toss hot wings with olive oil mixture to coat.

Nutrition Facts Per Serving:

1180.6 calories; protein 20.8g 42% DV; carbohydrates 0.3g; fat 123.1g 189% DV; cholesterol 58mg 19% DV; sodium 409.1mg 16% DV.

Caramelized Chicken Wings

Ingredients

1 cup water

½ cup white sugar

⅓ cup soy sauce

2 tablespoons peanut butter

1 tablespoon honey

2 teaspoons wine vinegar

1 tablespoon minced garlic

12 eaches large chicken wings, tips removed and wings cut in half at joint

1 teaspoon sesame seeds, or to taste

Directions

Step 1

In an electric skillet or a large skillet over medium heat, mix together the water, sugar, soy sauce, peanut butter, honey, wine vinegar, and garlic until smooth and the sugar has dissolved. Place the wings into the sauce, cover, and simmer for 30 minutes. Uncover and simmer until the wings are tender and the sauce has thickened, about 30 more minutes, spooning sauce over wings occasionally. Sprinkle with sesame seeds.

Nutrition Facts Per Serving:

528.5 calories; protein 36.2g 72% DV; carbohydrates 22.4g 7% DV; fat 32.4g 50% DV; cholesterol 141.7mg 47% DV; sodium 962.5mg 39% DV.

Simple Grilled Lamb Chops

Ingredients

¼ cup distilled white vinegar

2 teaspoons salt

½ teaspoon black pepper

1 tablespoon minced garlic

1 onion, thinly sliced

2 tablespoons olive oil

2 pounds lamb chops

Directions

Step 1

Mix together the vinegar, salt, pepper, garlic, onion, and olive oil in a large resealable bag until the salt has dissolved. Add lamb, toss until coated, and marinate in refrigerator for 2 hours.

Step 2

Preheat an outdoor grill for medium-high heat.

Step 3

Remove lamb from the marinade and leave any onions on that stick to the meat. Discard any remaining marinade. Wrap the exposed ends of the bones with aluminum foil to keep them from burning. Grill to desired doneness, about 3 minutes per side for medium. The chops may also be broiled in the oven about 5 minutes per side for medium.

Nutrition Facts Per Serving:

519 calories; protein 25g 50% DV; carbohydrates 2.3g 1% DV; fat 44.8g 69% DV; cholesterol 112mg 37% DV; sodium 861mg 34% DV.

Dirty Piggy-Back Lamb

Ingredients

2 tablespoons olive oil

1 (8 ounce) package sliced fresh mushrooms

8 slices bacon

4 raw chop with refuse, 120 g; (blank) 4.225 ounces lamb blade chops

1 teaspoon cracked black peppercorns

1 pinch seasoned salt to taste

Directions

Step 1

Preheat a grill for high heat.

Step 2

While the grill warms up, heat the olive oil in a large skillet over medium heat. Add the mushrooms; cook and stir until tender. Set aside.

Step 3

Season the bacon slices with pepper, and place them on the grill. Cook bacon until crisp, turning once, then set aside. Season the lamb chops with seasoned salt, and place them on the grill. Cook to your desired degree of doneness, about 3 minutes per side for medium.

Step 4

Serve each chop with two slices of bacon over it, and top with the sliced mushrooms.

Nutrition Facts Per Serving:

351.3 calories; protein 22.8g 46% DV; carbohydrates 2.4g 1% DV; fat 27.7g 43% DV; cholesterol 76.7mg 26% DV; sodium 530.7mg 21% DV.

Herbed Lamb Chops

Ingredients

½ cup olive oil

½ cup red wine vinegar

¼ cup white wine

2 tablespoons lemon juice

2 cloves garlic, peeled and minced

¼ cup minced onion

1 teaspoon dried tarragon

1 teaspoon chopped fresh parsley

1 teaspoon black pepper

4 raw chop with refuse, 120 g; (blank) 4.225 ounces lamb chops

Directions

Step 1

In a large, nonreactive container, blend the olive oil, red wine vinegar, white wine, lemon juice, garlic, and onion. Season with tarragon, parsley, and pepper. Place lamb chops in the mixture. Cover, and marinate in the refrigerator about 2 hours.

Step 2

Preheat an outdoor grill for high heat, and lightly oil grate.

Step 3

Grill lamb chops on the prepared grill 5 minutes per side, to an internal temperature of 145 degrees F (63 degrees C). Discard remaining marinade.

Nutrition Facts Per Serving:

565.8 calories; protein 15.9g 32% DV; carbohydrates 5.2g 2% DV; fat 52.4g 81% DV; cholesterol 70.3mg 23% DV; sodium 56mg 2% DV.

Lamb Chops with Balsamic Reduction

Ingredients

¾ teaspoon dried rosemary

¼ teaspoon dried basil

½ teaspoon dried thyme

1 pinch salt and pepper to taste

4 raw chop with refuse, 120 g; (blank) 4.225 ounces lamb chops (3/4 inch thick)

1 tablespoon olive oil

¼ cup minced shallots

⅓ cup aged balsamic vinegar

¾ cup chicken broth

1 tablespoon butter

Directions

Step 1

In a small bowl or cup, mix together the rosemary, basil, thyme, salt and pepper. Rub this mixture onto the lamb chops on both sides. Place them on a plate, cover and set aside for 15 minutes to absorb the flavors.

Step 2

Heat olive oil in a large skillet over medium-high heat. Place lamb chops in the skillet, and cook for about 3 1/2 minutes per side for medium rare, or continue to cook to your desired doneness. Remove from the skillet, and keep warm on a serving platter.

Step 3

Add shallots to the skillet, and cook for a few minutes, just until browned. Stir in vinegar, scraping any bits of lamb from the bottom of the skillet, then stir in the chicken broth. Continue to cook and stir over medium-high heat for about 5 minutes, until the sauce has reduced by half. If you don't, the sauce will be runny and not good. Remove from heat, and stir in the butter. Pour over the lamb chops, and serve.

Nutrition Facts Per Serving:

254.5 calories; protein 14.6g 29% DV; carbohydrates 5g 2% DV; fat 19.3g 30% DV; cholesterol 63.9mg 21% DV; sodium 70.4mg 3% DV.

Fresh Tomato Salsa

Ingredients

3 medium whole (2-3/5" dia) (blank)s tomatoes, chopped

½ cup finely diced onion

5 eaches serrano chiles, finely chopped

½ cup chopped fresh cilantro

1 teaspoon salt

2 teaspoons lime juice

Directions

Step 1

In a medium bowl, stir together tomatoes, onion, chili peppers, cilantro, salt, and lime juice. Chill for one hour in the refrigerator before serving.

Nutrition Facts Per Serving:

51.5 calories; protein 2.1g 4% DV; carbohydrates 9.7g 3% DV; fat 0.2g; cholesterolmg; sodium 592.1mg 24% DV.

CONCLUSION

We all have different body systems and our reactions to dietary plans may be different, however it is imperative that we study and know what works best for us. The low residue diet has been prescribed to assist in the healing of the colon. It is also used on a temporary basis to prepare for procedures. Ensuring diet is low in fiber and fat. Milk and milk products should be avoided in people with diarrhea and/or lactose intolerance. Nutritional supplements that are low in residue and are lactose free, such as Ensure, Ensure Plus, and Sustacal, can be added to the low residue diet if additional calories and/or protein are needed.

Also know that following the diet temporarily, helps to improve symptoms and make eating more enjoyable and don't hesitate to ask your physician if he knows a nutritionist who can help make sure your diet is right for you and let you know if you need to take supplements.

Printed in Great Britain
by Amazon